BARTTER SYNDROME DISEASE DIET COOKBOOK

A Comprehensive Guide To Empowers Patients With Delicious Recipes, Kitchen Essentials, And Expert Advice For Managing Symptoms And Thriving Long-Term.

Dr. Holmgren Alfred

For those negotiating the complications of Bartter Syndrome, a rare but serious disorder affecting kidney function, the "Bartter Syndrome Diet Cookbook: Expert Guidance" is an invaluable resource.

Readers will discover a wealth of culinary knowledge and useful guidance within its pages, specifically catered to the nutritional requirements of those who are treating this condition.

Offering more than simply recipes provides a thorough understanding of Bartter Syndrome and how eating may be a key factor in managing the condition. It is a source of hope and empowerment.

The book's in-depth exploration of the subtleties of Bartter Syndrome, which gives readers a complete grasp of its causes, symptoms, and possible complications, is among its most captivating aspects.

Armed with important insights, this foundational knowledge enables people to take charge of their health journey. Furthermore, the focus on dietary recommendations highlights the significant influence nutrition can have on symptom relief and general well-being.

The cookbook is more useful than just a collection of recipes. It explores the practical side of keeping a kitchen that is conducive to Bartter Syndrome, from choosing the appropriate culinary utensils to stocking the pantry with necessities.

Even the busiest people can easily incorporate nutrient-dense meals into their daily routines with careful planning and preparation advice.

There are a ton of delicious recipes on its pages for breakfast, lunch, dinner, snacks, and even decadent desserts. Every recipe has been carefully designed to satisfy the palate while also adhering to the nutritional requirements specific to Bartter Syndrome. With recipes ranging from nutrient-dense smoothies to delectable dinners and cool drinks, the cookbook guarantees that people may enjoy a wide variety of foods without sacrificing their health.

The book also offers helpful advice on how to handle Bartter Syndrome when dining out and handling special occasions, so it's not just limited to the kitchen. With meal planning techniques, frugal shopping advice, and motivational success stories, it gives readers the resources they need to succeed over the long term on their path to optimum health.

Essentially, the "Bartter Syndrome Diet Cookbook: Expert Guidance" is more than just a cookbook; it's a source of empowerment that points people in the direction of a happier, better life even in the face of the obstacles that come with having Bartter Syndrome. It is a monument to the nutritional transformation that may occur when one embraces vitality and overcomes adversity, with its delicious cuisine and professional coaching.

The contents of the book "Bartter Syndrome Diet Cookbook with Expert Guidance" are solely for informational purposes. Since [Your Name], the book's author is not a licensed medical practitioner, its contents should not be construed as medical advice or used in place of expert medical diagnosis, consultation, or treatment.

Before implementing any dietary adjustments or making judgments regarding Bartter syndrome or any other medical issue covered in this book, readers should speak with a licensed healthcare provider.

Regarding the accuracy, comprehensiveness, dependability, or usefulness of the material supplied, the author makes no claims or guarantees. The reader assumes all risks when relying on the material in this book.

Any mention or reference to any person, thing, website, association, or other name in this book is purely informative and does not indicate that the author supports or is associated with it. The writer expressly disavows any affiliation or support for these organizations.

Moreover, the author disclaims all responsibility for any loss, harm, or damage resulting from using or depending on the information in this book.

Upon perusing this book, you yield any claims, damages, and other obligations against the author, publisher, and any affiliates arising from your use of or reliance on the material contained herein.

I appreciate your understanding.

CHAPTER 1
AN OVERVIEW OF BARRETT SYNDROME AND ITS NUTRITIONAL REQUIREMENTS

An uncommon hereditary condition called Bartter Syndrome is characterized by abnormalities in the kidney's capacity to reabsorb salt and chloride ions.

The kidneys' tubules, which are in charge of filtering and reabsorbing water and electrolytes, are the main organs affected by this illness. Due to these abnormalities, people with Bartter Syndrome lose a lot of water and salt in their urine, which can cause electrolyte imbalances, dehydration, and other related problems. The pediatrician Frederic Bartter, who initially described the syndrome in the 1960s, is honored by the syndrome's name. Based on the particular genetic alterations involved, Bartter Syndrome is categorized into numerous subtypes, the most prevalent of which are classic Bartter Syndrome and Gitelman Syndrome.

Overview of Bartter Syndrome: Polyuria (excessive urination), polydipsia (excessive thirst), muscle weakness, exhaustion, cravings for salt, and delays in a child's growth are just a few of the symptoms that this syndrome presents with. Depending on the Bartter Syndrome subtype, these symptoms might vary in severity and onset, although they usually appear during infancy or youth. Normal renal function and electrolyte balance are disrupted by the underlying genetic abnormalities that impact different ion channels and transporters in the kidney. As a result, Bartter Syndrome sufferers need lifetime care to minimize symptoms, avoid complications, and enhance their quality of life.

Summary of the Causes, Symptoms, and Complications Gene mutations encoding proteins involved in ion transport inside the kidney, specifically in the thick ascending limb of the loop of Henle, are the primary cause of Bartter Syndrome. Ion reabsorption is disrupted by mutations in genes such as SLC12A1, which codes for the Na-K-2Cl cotransporter, or KCNJ1, which codes for the renal outer medullary potassium channel. This results in the distinctive electrolyte abnormalities associated with Bartter Syndrome. Depending on the syndrome's subtype and severity, the clinical appearance might vary, although electrolyte abnormalities such as hypokalaemia (low potassium levels), metabolic alkalosis (high blood pH), and hypercalciuria (increased calcium excretion) are frequently seen.

Growth retardation, kidney stones, nephrocalcinosis (calcium deposits in the kidneys), and in extreme cases, renal failure, are all possible outcomes of untreated Bartter Syndrome.

The Role of Nutrition in Managing Bartter Syndrome: Adequate nutrition is essential to the overall care of people with Bartter Syndrome. Maintaining appropriate hydration and electrolyte balance is crucial due to the increased losses of sodium, chloride, potassium, and other electrolytes through the urine. This usually entails consuming foods high in potassium and salt to offset losses through urine and avoid electrolyte imbalances. Dietary modifications, however, must be customized to meet the unique requirements of each person, taking into consideration elements including age, the type of Bartter Syndrome, renal function, and the existence of comorbidities. Furthermore, careful monitoring of electrolyte levels via routine blood testing is necessary to prevent both excess and deficiency of important nutrients and to modify dietary recommendations accordingly.

Dietary Guidelines and Considerations: Optimising sodium, potassium, and fluid intake is a common strategy in the management of Bartter Syndrome to counteract electrolyte imbalance and urine losses. It's common knowledge that eating foods high in sodium, like processed meats, canned soups, and salted snacks, will raise the body's sodium levels. In a similar vein, meals high in potassium, such as leafy greens, potatoes, bananas, and oranges, can help restore potassium levels and avert hypokalemia. In order to meet their specific dietary needs, people with Bartter Syndrome must frequently consume certain items in appropriate quantities. On the other hand, overindulging in potassium or salt should be avoided as this might worsen cardiovascular problems such as edema and hypertension. Furthermore, in certain instances, nutritional supplements or pharmaceuticals may be recommended to address particular deficiencies or metabolic abnormalities linked to Bartter Syndrome. Overall, the best way to manage Bartter Syndrome and achieve long-term health outcomes is to follow a customized, well-balanced diet and have regular check-ups with medical professionals.

CHAPTER 2
BUILDING A BARTER SYNDROME-FRIENDLY KITCHEN

The first step in creating a kitchen that is Bartter Syndrome-Friendly is selecting pantry essentials that will help you properly manage the symptoms of the condition. To reduce symptoms and enhance general health, people with Bartter Syndrome, a rare genetic renal disease marked by electrolyte imbalances and kidney malfunction, must follow a diet high in certain nutrients and low in others. Keeping the pantry stocked with appropriate ingredients serves as the foundation for this project. Important mainstays include foods high in potassium, like sweet potatoes, spinach, and bananas, which help prevent the potassium wasting that is linked to Bartter syndrome.

Furthermore, consuming foods high in calcium, such as dairy products or fortified plant-based substitutes, helps to sustain calcium levels, which are important for bone health even in the face of the syndrome's renal difficulties. Moreover, foods high in magnesium, such as nuts, seeds, and whole grains, are critical for maintaining nerve and muscle function, which is necessary for those with Bartter Syndrome. People with this illness must control blood pressure and fluid balance, therefore choosing low-sodium substitutes and avoiding high-sodium processed foods. Incorporating protein sources such as fish, poultry, lentils, and lean meats guarantees a sufficient intake of protein while reducing levels of potassium and phosphorus, which can worsen symptoms in those with Bartter Syndrome.

Through careful selection and stocking the pantry with these Bartter-friendly items, people can optimize their health outcomes and better manage their condition.

Meal preparation is improved and dietary adherence is supported when the kitchen is furnished with necessary tools and equipment specific to the needs of individuals with Bartter Syndrome, in addition to stocking the pantry with appropriate items. A high-quality blender is a necessary kitchen item for Bartter Syndrome sufferers to prepare nutrient-rich smoothies and purees, which make it simpler for the body to absorb and digest vital nutrients. Purchasing an accurate digital food scale also helps with portion control, which is important when it comes to keeping an eye on sodium and potassium consumption, which is necessary for properly treating the symptoms of Bartter Syndrome. Additionally, cooking with a range of cookware—including steam baskets, nonstick pans, and slow cookers—allows people to make meals with little additional oil or sodium, maintaining the food's nutritional value while boosting flavor.

Additionally, having utensils like silicone spatulas and ladles on hand keeps non-stick surfaces from being scratched, extending the life of cookware that is necessary for meal preparation that is pleasant to people with Bartter Syndrome. Those who manage Bartter Syndrome can simplify food preparation, follow dietary recommendations, and ultimately enhance their general health and well-being by stocking their kitchen with these necessary appliances.

For those coping with Bartter Syndrome, efficient meal planning and preparation techniques are essential to ensuring adequate nutrition, controlling symptoms, and advancing long-term health.

Meal preparation in advance enables careful consideration of component selection, portion control, and nutrient balance about the dietary requirements of Bartter Syndrome. When meal planning, it is important to prioritize moderation and diversity to minimize the danger of excessive consumption of potassium, sodium, or phosphorus, which can worsen symptoms in individuals with Bartter Syndrome and prevent nutrient deficiencies. Furthermore, using meal prep strategies like batch cooking and portioning meals into individual servings makes it easier to follow nutritional requirements and ensures convenience, especially during hectic times or while dealing with symptoms that impair movement or energy. Additionally, seeking the advice of a qualified dietitian with expertise in renal nutrition can offer tailored direction and assistance in meal planning, guaranteeing customized nutritional approaches that complement the objectives of managing Bartter Syndrome. Meal planning techniques that put convenience, variety, and adequate nutrition first help people with Bartter Syndrome stick to their diets, control their symptoms as best they can, and live better overall.

CHAPTER 3
RECIPES FOR BREAKFAST

When creating breakfast meals for people with Bartter syndrome, it is critical to give priority to nutrient-dense options that support general health and well-being in addition to providing nourishment. A healthy breakfast is essential to promote proper body function given the physiological obstacles associated with Bartter syndrome, including electrolyte imbalances and renal abnormalities. A wide range of foods that are abundant in important vitamins, minerals, and macronutrients including protein, carbs, and healthy fats make up nutrient-rich breakfast selections. Eating meals high in potassium, magnesium, calcium, and other electrolytes can assist promote electrolyte balance and correct possible shortages.

This is especially crucial for those with Bartter syndrome, since they may lose more of these minerals through urine. Lean protein sources, whole grains, fruits, and vegetables can also help to sustain energy levels and encourage satiety throughout the morning, which helps to maintain stable blood sugar levels and avoid crashes and spikes. People with Bartter syndrome can start their day on a healthy note and improve their general health and well-being by focusing on nutrient density in breakfast meals. For those with Bartter syndrome, who may experience dietary limitations and other health issues, simple and quick breakfast options come in rather handy on hectic mornings when time is of the essence. In addition to saving time, quick breakfast options guarantee that people with Bartter syndrome can still eat wholesome meals despite their busy schedules. Simple yet nourishing recipes that just take a few minutes to prepare, like yogurt parfaits, whole-grain toast with sliced fruit and nut butter, or overnight oats, may be included in this list. Breakfast preparation can also be streamlined by preparing items in advance and using time-saving kitchen tools like food processors or blenders. Simple breakfast solutions meet the practical needs of people with Bartter syndrome by emphasizing speed without sacrificing nutritional quality, allowing them to continue eating a balanced diet even when they are pressed for time.

Smoothies and shakes that are suitable for people with Bartter syndrome provide a tasty and adaptable breakfast choice by combining vital nutrients into a form that is easy to ingest. Shakes and smoothies can be made with components that promote electrolyte balance and general health, tailored to the dietary requirements and tastes of people with Bartter syndrome. For instance, leafy greens high in magnesium, like kale or bananas, calcium-fortified dairy or plant-based milk, and fruits high in potassium, like bananas or oranges, might help address any nutrient deficits typically linked with Bartter syndrome. Adding protein sources like nut butter, Greek yogurt, or protein powder can also improve satiety and promote the health of your muscles. Additionally, using naturally sweet items like honey or berries might quell cravings without the need for extra sweets, which could be harmful to people who have Bartter syndrome. Bartter-friendly smoothies and shakes enable people with Bartter syndrome to start their day with a tasty and nutritious meal that fits their specific dietary needs and health goals by providing a quick and nutrient-dense breakfast choice.

CHAPTER 4
ENTREES FOR LUNCH AND DINNER

Within the framework of the "Bartter Syndrome Diet Cookbook," the Lunch and Dinner Entrees section offers a range of culinary selections catered to the unique dietary requirements and inclinations of those who are managing Bartter syndrome. This is an essential part of the cookbook; it has a wide range of recipes that are intended to satisfy both your hunger and your sense of taste buds, all the while following the dietary recommendations that are required to effectively manage the symptoms associated with Bartter syndrome.

The Lunch and Dinner Entrees section is centered around protein-rich main dishes that meet the dietary needs of people with Bartter syndrome, who may need to consume larger amounts of protein. Lean meats, chicken, fish, lentils, and tofu are just a few of the nutritious and easily digestible protein sources that are carefully chosen to include in these dishes. These main courses prioritize high-protein ingredients to support muscular health, encourage fullness, and contribute to a well-balanced diet.

Alongside the focus on protein, the cookbook features a lot of recipes that are vegetable-based, which emphasizes how important it is for people with Bartter syndrome to consume lots of vegetables in their diet. A wide variety of vegetables, such as colorful bell peppers, leafy greens, cruciferous vegetables, tomatoes, and root vegetables, are included in these dishes. These dishes maximize the nutritional potential of vegetables by providing a wealth of vital vitamins, minerals, antioxidants, and dietary fiber—all of which are crucial for maintaining optimum health and well-being.

For those with Bartter syndrome who may benefit from controlling their carbohydrate consumption, grain and starch alternatives are adaptable replacements for conventional carbohydrate sources in the Lunch and Dinner Entrees section. These substitutes cover a wide variety of possibilities, including gluten-free grains like sorghum and millet, as well as whole grains like quinoa, brown rice, and oats. Starchy vegetables—like sweet potatoes, butternut squash, and cauliflower—are also emphasized as wholesome substitutes for refined grains since they offer long-lasting energy and vital nutrients without raising blood sugar levels.

 Rich sauces and salad dressings that don't contain too much sodium are essential for improving the flavor and palatability of the dishes in the cookbook and for adhering to the dietary guidelines that are often advised for people with Bartter syndrome. using an emphasis on flavor, these sauces and dressings are made using herbs, spices, vinegar, citrus juices, and other aromatic ingredients to produce flavorful, robust dishes. Crucially, they are designed to utilize as little salt as possible, which lowers the possibility of electrolyte imbalances and promotes cardiovascular health in general.

Overall, the "Bartter Syndrome Diet Cookbook's Lunch and Dinner Entrees section embodies a holistic approach to nutritional support and culinary innovation, giving people with Bartter syndrome the tools they need to enjoy satisfying meals while effectively managing their symptoms and promoting long-term well-being. Through the emphasis on protein-dense main courses, vegetable-based appetizers, starch and grain substitutes, and tasty dressings and sauces without added salt, this section enables people with Bartter syndrome to adopt a satisfying and health-conscious eating plan.

CHAPTER 5
SNACKS AND APPETIZERS

Options For Healthful Snacks:

It is crucial to keep a well-balanced diet in the context of Bartter syndrome, a rare genetic condition marked by renal tubular failure that results in electrolyte abnormalities. Snacking is essential for maintaining sufficient nourishment and controlling the condition's symptoms. Foods that are high in vital minerals like calcium, magnesium, and vitamin D and low in sodium, potassium, and chloride should be the main focus of healthy snack selections for those with Bartter syndrome. To avoid aggravating the gastrointestinal symptoms that people with Bartter syndrome frequently experience, these foods should also be readily digested.

Fresh fruits like apples, pears, and berries are common healthy snack alternatives that are good for people with Bartter syndrome because they are naturally low in potassium and sodium. Furthermore, raw veggies that don't cause electrolyte imbalances, such as bell peppers, cucumbers, and carrots, offer vital vitamins and minerals. Nuts and seeds, like walnuts, pumpkin seeds, and almonds, can be great providers of vitamins, healthy fats, and protein. Nonetheless, to reduce sodium consumption, it is imperative to choose unsalted kinds. Additionally, yogurt and cheese can be added to snacks to increase the amount of calcium consumed; however, people who have Bartter syndrome should be aware of the potassium content and choose low-potassium choices.

When choosing healthy snack options for people with Bartter syndrome, frequency of consumption and portion sizes should be taken into account.

Snacks should be taken in moderation to avoid taxing the kidneys and escalating electrolyte imbalances. Additionally, seeking advice from a medical expert or registered dietitian with expertise in renal nutrition might yield customized recommendations catered to the unique requirements and dietary limitations of people with Bartter syndrome.

Bartter-Friendly Snacks For Events And Get-Togethers:

For those with Bartter syndrome, navigating social events and parties can be difficult, especially when it comes to making dietary decisions that could worsen symptoms or upset electrolyte balance. But it is possible to make appetizers that are both crowd-pleasing and Bartter-friendly with a little forethought and imagination. Sodium, potassium, and chloride-free foods should be the main focus of barter-friendly appetizers, which should also offer a variety of flavors and textures to suit a wide range of palates.

A crudité plate with a variety of fresh veggies, such as cherry tomatoes, snap peas, and radishes, plus a tasty hummus or yogurt-based dip is one idea for appetizers that go well with Bartters. This gives guests a refreshing and nourishing choice in addition to a visually pleasing and colorful display. Furthermore, low-potassium snacks or skewers made with lean protein (like shrimp or chicken) and low-potassium ingredients (like cucumber and melon) can be a favorite at gatherings and yet be safe for those with Bartter syndrome.

Small servings of baked or grilled meats, like turkey meatballs or chicken skewers, can be paired with vegetable-based sides like roasted Brussels sprouts or cauliflower nibbles for those looking for heartier options. These appetizers maintain their nutritional value and taste while providing a filling and high-protein choice.

Moreover, without depending on high-sodium seasonings or sauces, the flavor of Bartter-friendly appetizers can be improved by adding herbs, spices, and citrus flavors.

It is crucial to discuss dietary needs and preferences with the host or hostess when organizing Bartter-friendly appetizers for get-togethers and parties to make sure that appropriate options are available. To avoid uncomfortable symptoms during social gatherings, people with Bartter syndrome should also watch their electrolyte intake and portion sizes.

Bartter-friendly appetizers can help ensure that every guest has a great and pleasurable dining experience by emphasizing nutrient-dense products and inventive culinary techniques.

Carrying Snacks For A Move:

For those with Bartter syndrome, eating on the go can be difficult because convenience frequently means sacrificing nutritional value. Convenient and Bartter-friendly portable snacks can help people properly manage their symptoms while fitting into their busy lifestyles. Considerations like ease of carrying, shelf stability, and nutrient composition should be made when choosing portable snacks for those with Bartter syndrome.

Pre-packaged trail mix or nut and seed blends are a handy option for on-the-go snacking because they offer a portable supply of protein, healthy fats, and vital minerals. To reduce sodium intake and avoid electrolyte imbalances, it's crucial to select unsalted versions. Comparably, single servings of dried fruits like figs, raisins, and apricots can provide natural sweetness and dietary fiber in addition to being easy snacks.

If you're more of a savory snacker, single-serve servings of low-sodium cheese or nut butter combined with rice cakes or whole-grain crackers can make for a filling and portable snack. Moreover, homemade energy balls or protein bars including nuts, dates, and oats can be easily transported and prepared ahead of time for consumption while on the go. These snacks enhance energy levels and encourage satiety throughout the day by providing a balance of fats, proteins, and carbohydrates.

Including transportable fruits like oranges, bananas, or apples in snack selections can also offer a convenient and wholesome way to get your fill of vitamins and minerals on the road. Furthermore, for those with Bartter syndrome, portion sizes of Greek yogurt or cottage cheese topped with fruit might provide a quick and high-protein snack alternative. With planning and nutrient-dense snack choices that meet dietary guidelines, people with Bartter syndrome can effectively control their symptoms while maintaining a healthy and invigorated state of mind throughout the day.

CHAPTER 6
<u>SALADS AND SIDES</u>

For those with Bartter syndrome, colorful salads made with Bartter-friendly vegetables are a tasty and nutritious option. An uncommon genetic condition called Bartter syndrome is defined by abnormalities in the kidney's capacity to reabsorb specific electrolytes, which can cause abnormalities in the body's fluid and electrolyte levels. Salads high in potassium, magnesium, and other vital minerals become especially important when treating Bartter syndrome, since maintaining adequate electrolyte balance and hydration is crucial. A colorful assortment of fruits and vegetables, including bell peppers, avocados, tomatoes, cucumbers, and leafy greens, are frequently included in these salads. These components add to the dish's aesthetic appeal while also offering vital vitamins and minerals that are needed for general health and well-being. Additionally, using Bartter-friendly foods guarantees that people with this illness can savor their meals without aggravating their symptoms or sacrificing their dietary intake.

The Bartter syndrome diet would not be complete without delectable vegetable side dishes, which offer a wide variety of tastes and textures as well as vital elements to promote general health. When it comes to making sure that people with Bartter syndrome have enough potassium, magnesium, and other electrolytes, which are necessary for maintaining correct fluid balance and muscular function, vegetable side dishes are a critical component. Rich in vitamins, minerals, and antioxidants, vegetables including spinach, kale, broccoli, carrots, and sweet potatoes are frequently used as side dishes that are suitable for Bartters. People with Bartter syndrome can enjoy a wide range of flavors and culinary experiences while also improving the nutritional value of their meals by adding a variety of vegetables to their side dishes. Vegetable side dishes can also be made in a variety of ways, such as roasting, steaming, or sautéing, which gives meal preparation and planning flexibility and inventiveness.

For those with Bartter syndrome, whole grain substitutes for traditional sides provide a wholesome and fulfilling way to enhance meals while fostering the best possible health and well-being. Whole grains are a great way to replace refined grains in the Bartter syndrome diet since they are high in fiber, complex carbs, and necessary nutrients. Examples of these grains are quinoa, brown rice, barley, and farro. Whole grains maintain their nutritional integrity, offering long-lasting energy and supporting digestive health, in contrast to refined grains, which go through processing that depletes them of their inherent fiber and nutrient content. Including whole grain substitutes with classic side dishes like bread, pasta, and rice improves the meal's nutritional profile and helps with blood sugar regulation and weight control—two factors that are crucial for people with Bartter syndrome. In addition, there are numerous delectable methods to serve whole grains, such as salads, side dishes, or pilafs, which promote culinary creativity and adaptability in the planning and preparation of meals. People with Bartter syndrome can eat tasty, nourishing meals that promote their general health and well-being by selecting whole-grain substitutes.

CHAPTER 7
TREATS AND DESSERTS

Desserts and treats are important to take into account while managing fumarate-deficient nutrition since they not only help to satiate cravings but also help to maintain a balanced diet that promotes overall health. Desserts and pastries can be quite difficult for people who have fumarate deficiency since they have to watch how much sodium they eat and make sure the components they use fit into their diet. However, it is feasible to enjoy delectable sweet sweets while following the required dietary requirements if you prepare ahead and use your imagination.

Dessert alternatives low in sodium: Cutting back on sodium is an important part of managing fumarate insufficiency because too much sodium can make symptoms worse and lead to complications.

Therefore, to satiate their sweet tooth without jeopardizing their health, people with fumarate insufficiency need to look for low-sodium dessert options. Desserts that are low in sodium usually use naturally low-sodium ingredients or replace high-sodium ingredients with healthier ones. Fresh fruits, which are naturally high in vitamins and antioxidants and low in salt, like berries, apples, and citrus fruits, are frequently used as part of diet plans. Using unsalted nuts, seeds, and whole grains can also enhance the flavor and texture of desserts without raising the sodium content. Additionally, erythritol, stevia, and monk fruit are some substitute sweeteners that can be used to lessen the total amount of sugar in sweets without sacrificing sweetness.

 Fruit-based desserts: Fruits are a great choice for people who are fumarate deficient and are looking for a wholesome and tasty dessert substitute. Fruits provide a wealth of vitamins, minerals, and dietary fiber that promote general health and well-being in addition to being naturally low in salt. Desserts made with fruit can be as basic as fruit salads and skewers or as complex as fruit tarts, sorbets, and compotes. People can enjoy sweet treats without adding sugar or high-sodium components by utilizing the inherent sweetness of fruits. Fruits also work well with a variety of cooking methods, such as baking, grilling, and poaching, opening up countless choices for dessert preparation. Desserts that are tasty and distinctive and satisfy dietary restrictions and personal tastes can be created by experimenting with different combinations of fruits, spices, and herbs.

Sweets produced with components that are Bartter-friendly: Although it may seem difficult to enjoy sweets while managing fumarate deficit, there are methods to savor flavors without sacrificing dietary constraints. People can support their health goals while satisfying their cravings for rich and indulgent flavors by carefully choosing Bartter-friendly items and combining them into treat recipes. Low-sodium substitutes for conventional high-sodium components, such as unsalted butter or margarine, low-sodium baking powder, and flavorings and extracts without sodium, are often included in barter-friendly products. People can also experiment with other grains and flours, including oat flour, coconut flour, or almond flour, which add flavor and texture to baked goods while providing nutritional advantages. Additionally, you may improve the richness and creaminess of desserts without using high-sodium items like cream or cheese by adding sources of healthy fats like avocado, almonds, and seeds. People who are fumarate deficient can enjoy a variety of decadent foods that meet their dietary requirements and tastes by being creative and innovative in the kitchen.

controlling the nutrition of fumarate insufficiency requires carefully thought-out choices for desserts and treats to maintain dietary limits while yet indulging in tasty and fulfilling sweets. People can enjoy delectable desserts that promote their general health and well-being by experimenting with Bartter-friendly ingredients, looking into low-sodium dessert substitutes, and adding fruits to dessert recipes. People who suffer from fumarate insufficiency can live long, healthy lives and satiate their sweet tooths sustainably by using creative cooking and thoughtful preparation.

CHAPTER 8
LIQUIDS

For those with Bartter syndrome, a rare genetic illness marked by the body's incapacity to reabsorb salt and chloride in the kidneys, beverages are an essential part of their diet and hydration regimen. Maintaining adequate hydration is crucial for controlling Bartter syndrome symptoms such as frequent urination, electrolyte abnormalities, and dehydration.

Thus, promoting the general health and well-being of Bartter patients requires the implementation of efficient hydration techniques. These tactics frequently entail drinking enough water and electrolytes throughout the day to make up for the increased losses of these elements through urine.

For Bartter patients, hydration therapies usually center on increasing fluid intake under close observation of electrolyte levels. Patients with Bartter syndrome must ensure that they consume enough of these beverages to replace the high amounts of sodium, potassium, and chloride that are lost through the urine. Although the best way to stay hydrated is through water, Bartter patients might also benefit from taking electrolyte-rich drinks, including sports drinks or oral rehydration treatments, to help keep their electrolyte balance in check. Including items high in water content, like fruits and vegetables, in the diet can also help maintain proper hydration levels.

Since too much salt can aggravate the symptoms and problems of Bartter syndrome, low-sodium beverage substitutes are essential to the nutritional management of the condition.

It is recommended that Bartter patients restrict their sodium consumption to avoid hypertension and fluid retention. Consequently, choosing low-sodium beverage substitutes is crucial for cutting back on sodium intake without sacrificing hydration levels. Unsweetened herbal teas, handmade fruit-infused water, and salt-free coconut water are a few examples of low-sodium drinks. For Bartter sufferers, these substitutes offer hydration without adding to sodium overload, improving symptom management and general wellness.

While following dietary guidelines and limits, inventive mocktail concoctions provide Bartter patients with a range of tasty and entertaining beverage options. Mocktails, also known as non-alcoholic cocktails, are made without the use of alcohol by combining a variety of fruits, herbs, and other tasty ingredients to make refreshing drinks. Mocktails offer a safe and entertaining substitute for Bartter sufferers who may need to restrict their intake of some beverages that contain alcohol or a lot of sugar. Fresh ingredients like berries, citrus fruits, mint, and sparkling water can be combined to make delectable mocktails that help Bartter patients meet their hydration objectives while also pleasing their palates. Bartter patients can customize mocktail recipes to suit their tastes and dietary requirements by experimenting with different flavor combinations and garnishes.

In conclusion, beverages are an essential part of the dietary therapy of Bartter syndrome. The goals of hydration methods are to preserve electrolyte balance and increase fluid consumption.

Bartter patients can reduce their salt consumption by using low-sodium beverage substitutes, and inventive mocktail recipes provide tasty, dietary-restricted options. Bartter patients can effectively manage their symptoms and enhance their general quality of life by implementing these concepts into their diet.

CHAPTER 9
SPECIAL OCCASION MENUS

People with Bartter Syndrome frequently struggle to enjoy special occasions while following dietary restrictions, as special cuisines customized to the theme or purpose of the event are common. When creating menus for special occasions, people with Bartter Syndrome must have their dietary requirements and preferences taken into account. Making meals low in potassium, sodium, and magnesium may be necessary because these electrolytes might cause issues for people who have Bartter Syndrome. Moreover, including foods high in potassium- and calcium-sparing diuretics, such as some fruits and vegetables, can support electrolyte balance maintenance while still offering palatable and fulfilling choices. Furthermore, it's critical to monitor portion sizes and meal time to avoid electrolyte imbalances, which have the potential to exacerbate Bartter Syndrome symptoms. Through careful collaboration with medical professionals and the use of tools like the Bartter Syndrome Diet Cookbook, people may design menus for special occasions that not only accommodate their dietary requirements but also enable them to fully partake in and enjoy celebratory activities.

Menus For Holidays And Celebrations:

Food is a major part of holidays and celebrations, which are both opportunities and difficulties for people with Bartter Syndrome. To ensure that people with Bartter Syndrome can fully engage in festivities while managing their illness properly, extensive thought and consideration go into creating holiday and celebration menus for them.

This may entail lowering the salt, potassium, and magnesium contents of classic holiday recipes to make them better suited for people with Bartter Syndrome. For instance, you can still produce delectable dishes without going overboard with your dietary limitations by using herbs and seasonings that don't include salt instead of salt, and by occasionally adding items high in potassium. Moreover, providing a range of options—such as salads, desserts produced with low-potassium ingredients, and protein-rich dishes—can offer people with Bartter Syndrome a varied and pleasurable dining experience during special occasions and festivities. Additionally, providing information to family members, guests, and the public regarding Bartter Syndrome and the dietary restrictions related to it can foster a welcoming and inclusive atmosphere where people feel secure in managing their condition while enjoying holidays with loved ones.

Having Bartter Syndrome Visitors:

It takes great preparation and thought to host visitors with Bartter Syndrome and make sure their dietary requirements are satisfied while still serving delectable and filling meals. It's crucial to get in touch with visitors who have Bartter Syndrome in advance to learn about their unique dietary needs and preferences. This could entail finding out about things like high-potassium or high-sodium foods that they should limit or avoid because of their condition. It's also critical to get knowledgeable about substitute ingredients and cooking techniques that can be employed to satisfy certain dietary requirements while still producing tasty and entertaining meals. When creating the menu, think about providing a range of options, such as low-potassium, low-sodium, and high-calcium dishes, to accommodate various dietary requirements. Giving dishes clear labels or descriptions can also make it easier for visitors with Bartter Syndrome to traverse the dinner and make wise decisions. Through these actions and consideration of their visitors' dietary requirements, hosts can establish a warm and inclusive eating environment for people with Bartter Syndrome, enabling them to savor delectable meals without jeopardizing their health.

Advice for Handling Bartter Syndrome When Eating Out:

People with Bartter Syndrome may have particular difficulties when dining out because they have to read menus and follow dietary guidelines. For those with Bartter Syndrome, eating out can still be pleasurable and fulfilling if they prepare ahead and exercise awareness. It is useful to do some advanced research on restaurants before going out to eat to determine which ones provide selections that are appropriate for people with Bartter Syndrome. Finding appropriate options is now made easier for patrons by the proliferation of eateries that offer nutritional information or cater to specific dietary requirements. To make sure that meals are served appropriately, it is also helpful to discuss specific dietary preferences and limits with restaurant staff. When placing your order, choose meals that are low in sodium, potassium, and magnesium and request any necessary substitutions or adjustments. To regulate quantities and steer clear of unidentified electrolyte sources, it could also be beneficial to ask for dressings, sauces, and condiments on the side. Lastly, pay attention to how much food you eat, listen to your body, and stop when you're full to avoid consuming too much electrolytes. People with Bartter Syndrome can enjoy eating out while efficiently managing their disease if they adhere to these guidelines and speak out for their nutritional needs.

CHAPTER 10
LONG-TERM SUCCESS STRATEGIES AND MEAL PLANNING

A key component of controlling Bartter syndrome, a rare genetic condition that impairs the kidneys' capacity to reabsorb specific electrolytes, is meal planning.

A well-balanced diet is generally necessary for Bartter syndrome sufferers to avoid electrolyte imbalances and properly control their symptoms. Weekly meal planning techniques are covered in detail in the "Bartter Syndrome Diet Cookbook" to assist patients and caregivers in meeting their nutritional needs. This entails putting together a weekly meal and snack schedule that accounts for the required intake of potassium, magnesium, and other electrolytes as well as sufficient hydration. Making preparations in advance helps people keep stable electrolyte levels and better regulate their nutritional intake, which reduces the likelihood of Bartter syndrome consequences.

Recognizing that adhering to a specific diet can occasionally be expensive, the cookbook also includes budget-friendly purchasing advice. This section offers helpful tips on how to purchase cheaply without sacrificing meal quality or nutritional content.

It might contain advice on how to shop in bulk, choose seasonal produce, use store coupons and discounts, and prioritize necessities while cutting back on frivolous spending. Families and people impacted by Bartter syndrome can lower their grocery expenses while maintaining access to the items needed to make healthful and filling meals by putting these recommendations into practice.

One of the main features of the "Bartter Syndrome Diet Cookbook" is recipe adaptation. Because nutritional demands can differ greatly between people with Bartter syndrome, the cookbook provides instructions on how to alter dishes to suit individual needs and preferences.

This could be changing the components to change the flavor, texture, or electrolyte levels. It could also entail using different cooking techniques to improve the food's digestibility or lower its sodium content.

The cookbook guarantees that people with Bartter syndrome can enjoy a varied and fulfilling range of meals without compromising their nutritional goals or health results by enabling users to modify recipes according to their particular dietary restrictions and preferences.

Testimonials and success stories provide motivating illustrations of tenacity and sustained success in controlling Bartter syndrome with dietary changes.

These stories present first-hand accounts of people who, by following the dietary guidelines provided in the cookbook, overcame obstacles, enhanced their quality of life, and saw improvements in their health.

Through telling these tales, the cookbook not only inspires and motivates readers but also demonstrates how successful the suggested tactics are at fostering long-term well-being and symptom management.

In addition to promoting a sense of belonging and solidarity among those impacted by Bartter syndrome, success stories, and testimonies also serve to create a supportive environment in which people may share their experiences and exchange views to promote mutual learning and development.

CONCLUSION

For those with Bartter syndrome and their families, the "Bartter Syndrome Diet Cookbook" is an extensive and priceless resource. With a focus on meal planning, frugal shopping advice, recipe modification, and success stories, the cookbook offers helpful direction and motivation for symptom management and long-term success.

The cookbook provides readers with the knowledge and resources they need to take charge of their dietary management, maximize their nutritious intake, and improve their general quality of life.

It does this by energizing readers with mouthwatering recipes, kitchen necessities, and professional guidance. For those with Bartter syndrome and those who care for them, the "Bartter Syndrome Diet Cookbook" provides a comprehensive approach to nutritional support and a path toward resilience, health, and overall well-being.